ALL YOU NEED TO KNOW ABOUT THE KETOGENIC DIET FOR PEDIATRIC DRUG-RESISTANT EPILEPSY

USER MANUAL FOR PARENTS AND CAREGIVERS

SOMA BASU

HEMAMALINI A. J.

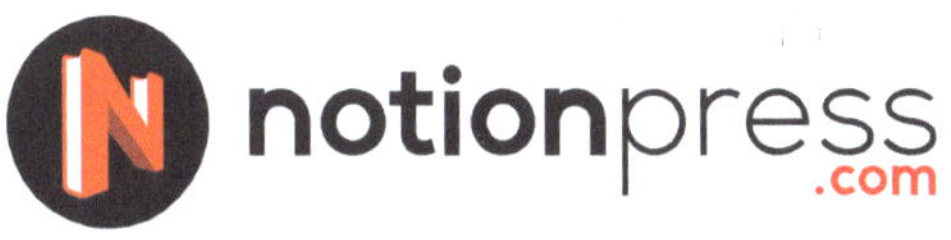

DISCLAIMER

The information provided in this book is intended for educational and informational purposes only. It is not meant to replace personalized medical advice, diagnosis, or treatment provided by qualified healthcare professionals. Always seek the advice of your child's pediatric neurologist, and a certified keto dietitian who has done his/her expertise in the ketogenic diet before making any changes to your child's medical treatment or dietary plan.

While every effort has been made to ensure the accuracy and completeness of the information contained herein, the author and publisher assume no responsibility for errors, omissions, or outcomes resulting from the use of this information. Each child's situation is unique, and medical decisions should always be made in consultation with treating team who are familiar with your child's individual needs.

The ketogenic diet is a medically prescribed therapy that should only be undertaken under the supervision and guidance of a healthcare team experienced in its use for epilepsy management. Never disregard professional medical advice or delay seeking treatment because of something you have read in this book.

By reading this book, you acknowledge that you are responsible for consulting with appropriate healthcare professionals regarding the information presented and for making your own healthcare decisions.

ABOUT THE BOOK

"All You Need to Know About the Ketogenic Diet for Pediatric Drug-Resistant Epilepsy" is a comprehensive, compassionate guide designed for parents navigating one of the toughest challenges: managing drug resistant epilepsy when anti seizure medications are not enough. This book breaks down the science behind the ketogenic diet, offers practical tips for everyday life, and provides emotional support for families walking this difficult road. From meal planning and medical monitoring to handling peer pressure and managing parental stress, this resource empowers caregivers with the knowledge, tools, and encouragement needed to help thier child thrive. Clear, accessible, and heartfelt, it is a must-have companion for anyone considering or already following the ketogenic diet for epilepsy treatment.

CONTENTS

Epilepsy is one of the most challenging neurological conditions that can affect children, and when seizures persist despite multiple anti-seizure medications — what we call drug-resistant epilepsy (DRE) — the burden on the child and family can be immense. In

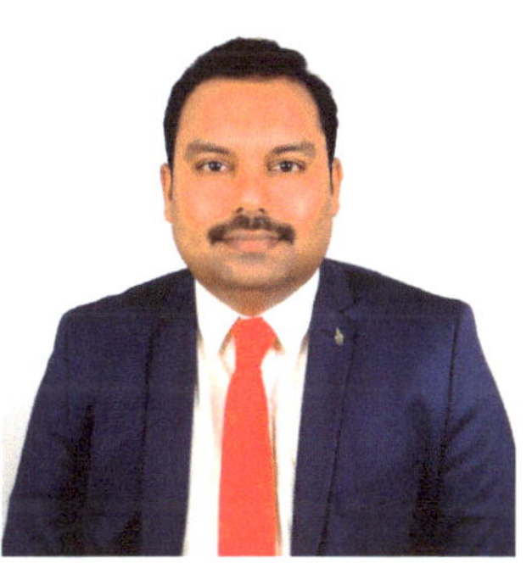

such cases, the ketogenic diet, a scientifically proven medical nutrition therapy, offers a beacon of hope.

As a pediatric neurologist and epileptologist, I have witnessed firsthand the remarkable impact the ketogenic diet can have on seizure control, cognition, and overall quality of life in children with DRE. Yet I also understand that starting and maintaining this diet — especially in the Indian context, with our rich and diverse food culture — can feel overwhelming for parents. The ketogenic diet is not simply a "low-carb" plan; it is a precision therapy, as critical to a child's treatment as any anti-seizure medication or surgical intervention.

This book, *All You Need to Know About the Ketogenic Diet for Pediatric Drug-Resistant Epilepsy*, has been thoughtfully written to empower Indian parents with accurate, practical, and compassionate guidance. It addresses not only the scientific foundations of the diet, but also the emotional, social, and cultural challenges that families often face. From meal planning to dealing with festivals, from monitoring progress to staying motivated — this resource offers a roadmap to help parents feel confident and supported every step of the way.

In India, where awareness about dietary therapies for epilepsy is still growing, a book like this is not just helpful; it is vital. I commend the authors for bridging the gap between medical science and daily family life in such an accessible manner.

To every parent reading this: you are not alone in your journey. With the right knowledge, determination, and support, it is possible to give your child the gift of better health and a brighter future. I hope this book serves as a trusted companion as you navigate the ketogenic path with courage and hope.

*– **Dr. Ranjith Kumar Manokaran***
Associate Professor,
Division of Pediatric Neurology and Epileptology
Senior Consultant Pediatric Neurologist & Epileptologist
Sri Ramachandra Institute of Higher Education and Research
Porur, Chennai, Tamil Nadu, India

PREFACE

When a child is diagnosed with drug-resistant epilepsy (DRE), life changes in an instant. Families are thrust into a world of uncertainty, searching for answers and solutions where standard treatments fall short. In this search, many discover a powerful, time-tested therapy that offers real hope: the ketogenic diet.

This book was born out of a deep understanding of the challenges, fears, and triumphs that parents experience when navigating the ketogenic journey. It is designed to be a practical, compassionate guide — one that explains the science behind the diet in clear terms, offers step-by-step support for day-to-day life, and addresses the emotional realities that come with caring for a child with DRE.

The ketogenic diet is not a fad or a trendy lifestyle choice; it is a serious, medically supervised therapy that has given countless children a new chance at a better, seizure-controlled life. However, following it can feel overwhelming without the right knowledge and encouragement. That's why this book exists — to empower you with the information, strategies, and confidence you need to succeed.

You will find chapters on everything from understanding how the diet works, meal planning and troubleshooting, to managing social situations and caring for your own emotional well-being. Wherever you are on this journey — just beginning, feeling stuck, or needing reassurance — this book is here to walk alongside you.

As you turn these pages, remember: you are not alone. There is hope, and with knowledge, support, and perseverance, the ketogenic diet can open doors to better health and a brighter future for your child.

Welcome to a path of resilience, healing, and renewed possibility.

– Soma Basu & Hemamalini A.J.

Chapter 1

UNDERSTANDING THE KETOGENIC DIET FOR PEDIATRIC DRUG-RESISTANT EPILEPSY

What is the Ketogenic Diet?

The ketogenic diet (often called "keto") is a high-fat, low-carbohydrate, and moderate-protein dietary therapy designed to shift the body's primary source of energy from carbohydrates (glucose) to fats (ketones). This shift in metabolism mimics the biochemical effects of fasting, which has long been known to reduce seizures.

When carbohydrate intake is drastically reduced, the liver begins to convert fat into ketones, which are then used by the brain as an alternative fuel source. In children with epilepsy, especially drug-resistant (refractory) epilepsy, this metabolic state of ketosis has been shown to have powerful anti-seizure effects.

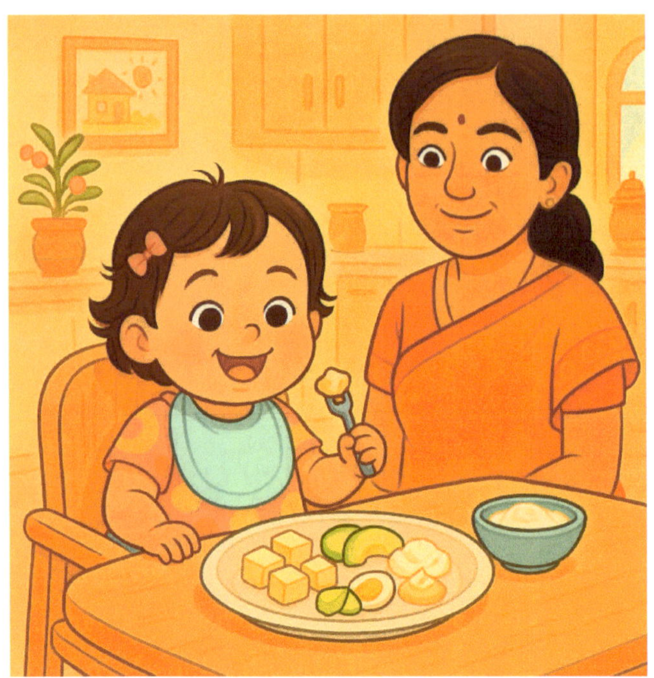

What is Drug Resistant Epilepsy?

Drug-resistant epilepsy is a condition where seizures persist despite treatment with two or more appropriate anti-seizure medications.

What is Ketosis?

A normal high-carbohydrate diet provides the brain with glucose as its main source of energy. However, in people with epilepsy, glucose metabolism may not work properly, and this can make brain cells more excitable, increasing the risk of seizures. In contrast, the ketogenic diet is very low in carbohydrates and high in fats, forcing the body to produce ketone bodies from fat for energy instead of relying on glucose.

When the brain uses ketones, neurons become less excitable, which helps reduce seizure activity. Ketones also seem to protect brain cells, reduce inflammation, and boost the production of calming brain chemicals like GABA. Overall, while a high-carb diet might continue to fuel an overactive brain, the ketogenic diet changes the brain's energy source to something that helps stabilize and calm brain activity, making seizures less likely.

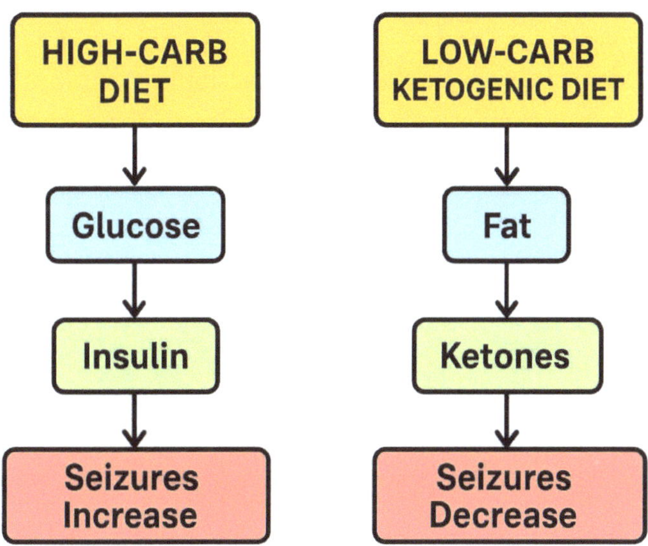

Historical Background

The ketogenic diet dates back to the 1920s when physicians at the Mayo Clinic observed that fasting helped control seizures. To mimic the effects of fasting, researchers developed the ketogenic diet. Although its use declined with the introduction of anti-seizure medications, it gained popularity again in the 1990s due to public success stories and has since become a standard therapeutic option for drug-resistant epilepsy.

How Does the Ketogenic Diet Help your child with Drug Resistant Epilepsy?

Though the exact mechanism is not fully understood, several theories explain its effectiveness:

1. Stabilizing Brain Energy

2. Reducing Excitatory Signals

3. Anti-inflammatory Effects

4. Improving Mitochondrial Function

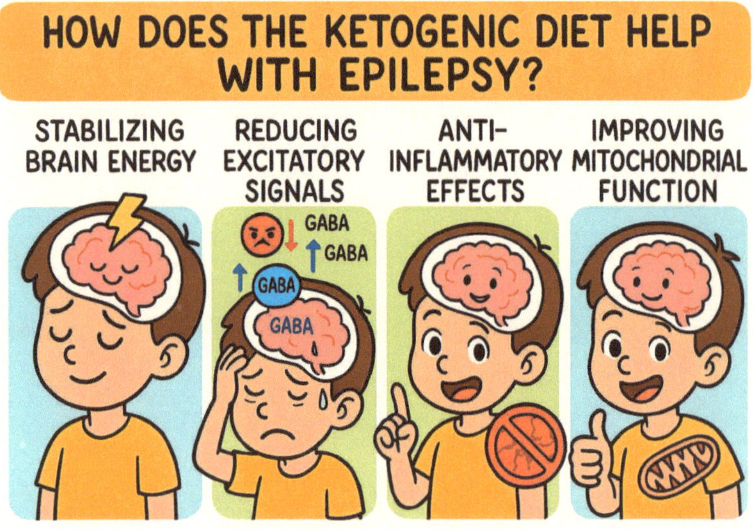

Role of Ketogenic Diet in Epilepsy

Types of Epilepsy That May Respond to Keto

The ketogenic diet is often recommended for children with drug-resistant epilepsy. It is especially beneficial in conditions such as

- Glucose Transporter Type 1 Deficiency Syndrome (GLUT1-DS)
- Pyruvate Dehydrogenase Deficiency (PDHD)
- Dravet Syndrome
- Lennox-Gastaut Syndrome (LGS)
- Doose Syndrome (Myoclonic-Astatic Epilepsy)
- Infantile Spasms (West Syndrome)
- Tuberous Sclerosis Complex
- Myoclonic Epilepsy of Infancy (MEI)
- FIRES (Febrile Infection-Related Epilepsy Syndrome)
- Rett Syndrome
- Mitochondrial Disorders (select cases)
- Idiopathic Generalized Epilepsy
- Focal Epilepsy with Structural Lesions
- Epilepsy of Unknown Etiology

How Effective Is It for your Child?

Clinical evidence suggests 50-60% of children see a >50% reduction in seizures and 20-30% may become seizure-free. It may also reduce or eliminate the need for anti-seizure medications.

Is It Safe for my Child?

Yes—when medically supervised. Potential side effects include constipation, nutrient deficiencies, kidney stones, elevated cholesterol, and slowed growth. These are manageable with proper monitoring.

Why Parents Should Consider the Ketogenic Diet for Drug Resistant Epilepsy?

The ketogenic diet offers a promising option for managing epilepsy in children, especially those with drug-resistant forms. With appropriate guidance and monitoring, it can lead to reduced seizures, improved development, and enhanced quality of life.

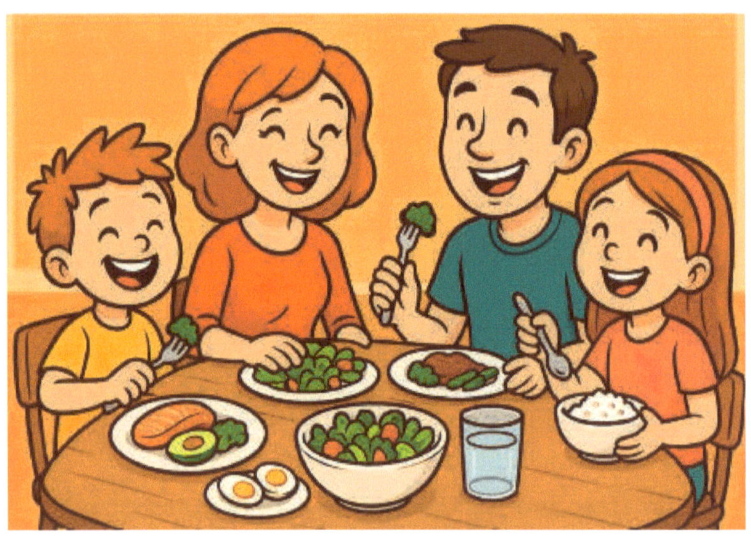

Family Enjoying Keto Meals

Chapter 2

WHAT YOU SHOULD KNOW AS A PARENT BEFORE STARTING

Starting the ketogenic diet for your child is a significant medical and lifestyle decision. This chapter aims to prepare you mentally, emotionally, and practically for what lies ahead. Before beginning the diet, parents need a clear understanding of the goals, challenges, medical protocols, and daily responsibilities involved. When done right, this therapeutic approach can bring life-changing results.

Unlike popular versions of the ketogenic diet for weight loss, the clinical ketogenic diet for epilepsy is a prescribed Medical Nutrition Therapy. It is not just "cutting carbs" or "eating healthy fats." Instead, it's a carefully crafted metabolic therapy that needs: strict nutritional ratios, daily monitoring, and ongoing medical supervision.

It's a Medical Nutrition Therapy—Not Just a Diet

You will need a team of specialists, typically including:

- A pediatric neurologist
- A certified ketogenic dietitian
- Possibly a clinical nurse, social worker, or psychologist

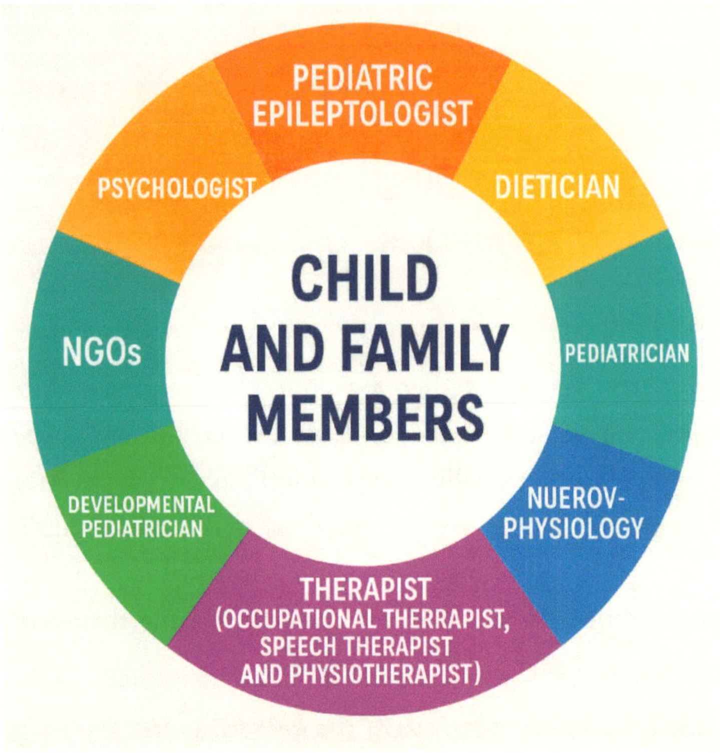

The Team

Not Every Child is a Candidate

Before starting the diet, your child will undergo a medical screening. The ketogenic diet is not safe for children with certain metabolic conditions, including:

- Fatty Acid Oxidation Disorders

- Carnitine deficiency

- Pyruvate carboxylase deficiency

- Some mitochondrial disorders

Your child may be a good candidate if he/she is having:

- Drug Resistant Epilepsy

- Metabolic condition like GLUT1 Deficiency or PDHD

- Specific epilepsy syndromes (e.g., Doose, Dravet)

- Seizures impact their development or daily functioning

You'll Need to Commit Fully

This is not a therapy you can "sort of" do—it requires 100% adherence to be effective. Expect it to take time to adjust. But many parents describe the process as difficult in the beginning but life-changing once it becomes routine.

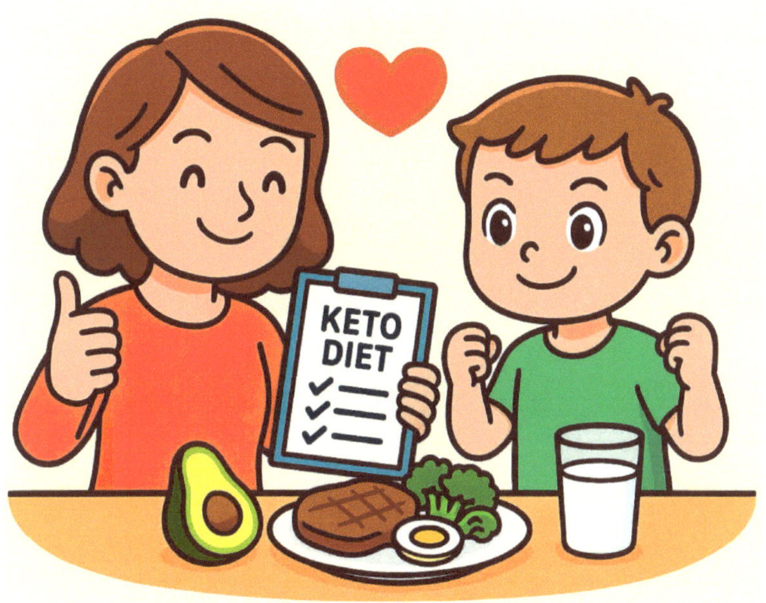

There Will Be an Adjustment Period

Most programs begin the diet gradually or through a hospital-based initiation under close observation. During the first few days, your child may feel tired or irritable, and you'll begin learning the essentials of meal planning and monitoring.

You'll Need to Learn New Skills

You'll learn how to:

- - Use a digital food scale
- - Read food labels
- - Track ketone levels
- - Recognize early signs of side effects
- - Communicate the diet's importance to others

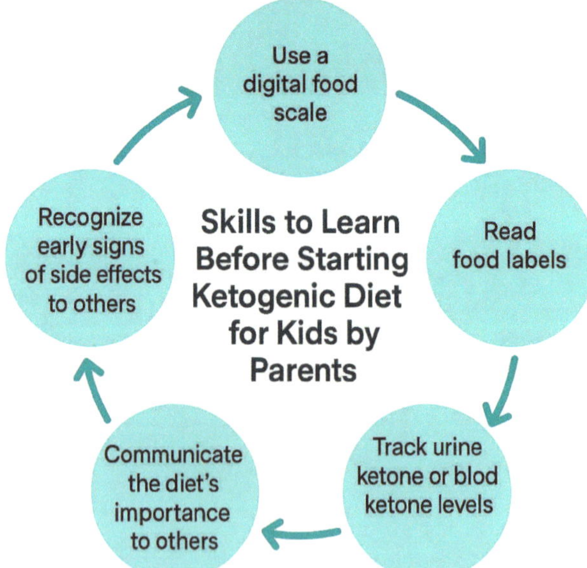

The Role of the Dietitian is Crucial

Your certified ketogenic dietitian will calculate your child's macronutrient ratio, design meal plans, monitor growth and labs, and help you make the diet sustainable.

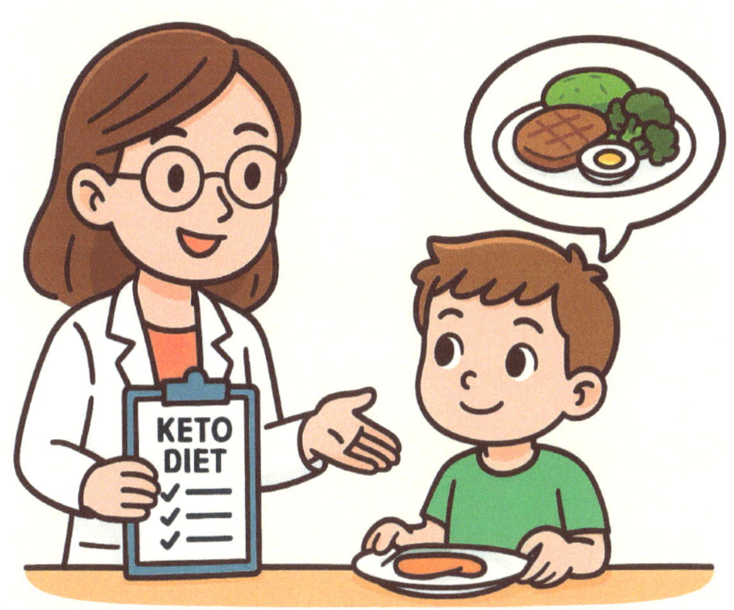

Understand the Potential Risks and Side Effects

Common Side Effects and How to Manage Them:

Side Effect	What to Watch For	Management
Constipation	Hard stools, infrequent bowel movements	High-fiber vegetables, hydration, laxatives
Low Blood Sugar	Fatigue, shakiness, confusion	Frequent glucose monitoring, glucose gel on hand

(Contd.)

Side Effect	What to Watch For	Management
Kidney Stones	Abdominal pain, blood in urine	Hydration, potassium citrate supplements
High Cholesterol	May be seen in blood tests	Often resolves, monitor with lipid panels
Nutrient Deficiencies	Weakness, poor growth, fatigue	Supplements (vitamins, calcium, selenium, etc.)
Slowed Growth	In rare cases	Regular growth tracking and calorie adjustments

❓ What is "Keto Flu"?

Keto flu is a group of temporary symptoms that some children (and adults) may experience when starting a ketogenic diet, particularly in the early days or first week. It's called a "flu" because the symptoms can feel similar to having the actual flu — but it's not caused by an infection.

When used in children with drug-resistant epilepsy, the ketogenic diet is a medically supervised high-fat, very low-carbohydrate, adequate-protein diet that changes the body's metabolism to use ketones for energy instead of glucose. As the body shifts into ketosis, the transition can lead to temporary side effects known collectively as keto flu.

Common Signs to Watch For

Symptom	Description
Tiredness	Child seems sleepy or low on energy
Irritability	More cranky or moody than usual
Nausea	Complains of feeling sick, may vomit
Stomach pain	Complains of tummy aches
Trouble focusing	Appears confused or distracted
Dry mouth or thirst	May be a sign of dehydration
Constipation	Trouble passing stools
Muscle cramps	Complains of pain in legs or arms

When Does It Happen?

- Usually starts within the first 2–5 days of starting the diet
- May last up to a week
- Not all children experience it

How Can You Help?

Action	What to Do
Keep them hydrated	Offer plenty of water throughout the day
Use electrolytes (if advised)	May be prescribed by the doctor to balance minerals

(Contd.)

Action	What to Do
🥣 Follow the dietitian's plan	Do not change meal portions or ingredients
😊 Allow rest	Let your child rest more than usual
🧍 Gentle activity	Light play may help boost energy slowly

⚠️ Call the Treating Team If

- Vomiting does not stop
- Your child is very sleepy or hard to wake
- Shows signs of confusion or poor coordination
- Has a fever
- Refuses to eat or drink
- You are worried — trust your instincts!

💬 Reassurance for Parents

Keto flu is usually mild and short-lived, and many children adjust quickly. The ketogenic diet, once established, can help reduce seizures in many cases. You're not alone — your child's medical team is here to guide you every step of the way.

Coping with Psychological Stress as a Parent on Ketogenic Journey

Parents managing a child's ketogenic diet for epilepsy often experience significant psychological stress. The constant vigilance required to maintain strict dietary control, the fear of seizures if the diet is broken, and the pressure of navigating social situations can lead to feelings of anxiety, guilt, and emotional exhaustion. Parents may also grieve the loss of spontaneity in family life and feel isolated from others who don't fully understand the medical necessity of the diet. To overcome this stress, it's crucial for parents to seek support — whether through counseling, support groups, or connecting with other families on similar journeys. Building a strong partnership with a knowledgeable medical team can also ease the burden, providing reassurance and guidance. Practicing self-care, setting realistic expectations, and celebrating small victories can help restore emotional balance, reminding parents that their efforts are not just about food but about giving their child the best possible chance for seizure control and a better quality of life.

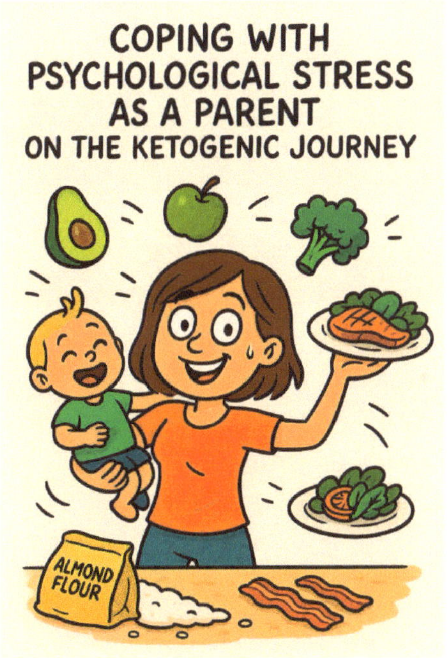

Set Your Goals and Expectations

Talk with your care team about goals like reducing seizure frequency or severity, reducing medications, or improving quality of life. You'll evaluate progress after about 3 months.

Are You Ready to Begin?

Before starting the ketogenic diet for epilepsy, be ready to commit to a structured routine, educate yourself, work with a team, monitor progress, and stay emotionally resilient.

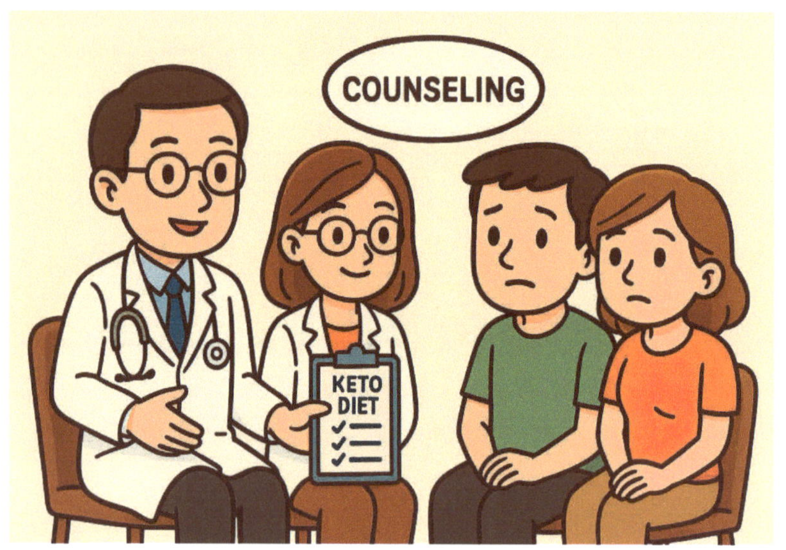

Chapter 3

GETTING STARTED WITH THE KETOGENIC DIET

Introduction

Beginning the ketogenic diet is a collaborative, structured process that involves thorough planning, education, and commitment. While the idea of "starting a diet" may sound as simple as changing what's on your child's plate, the therapeutic ketogenic diet requires careful preparation. This chapter walks you through what needs to happen before the first ketogenic meal is served.

Types of Ketogenic Diet

There are 4 types of ketogenic diet. They are -

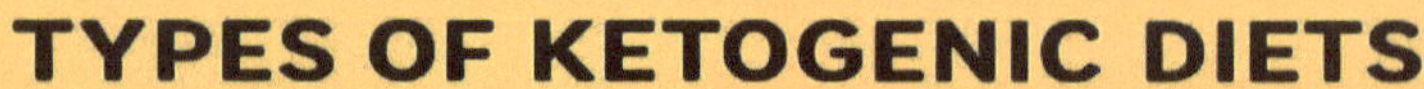

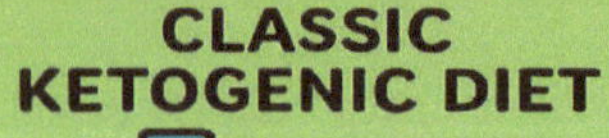

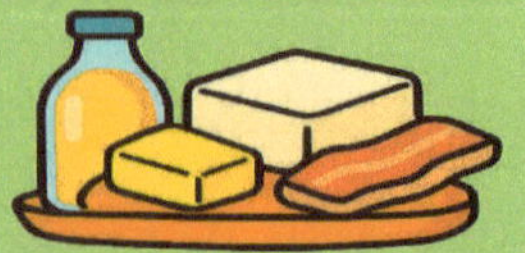

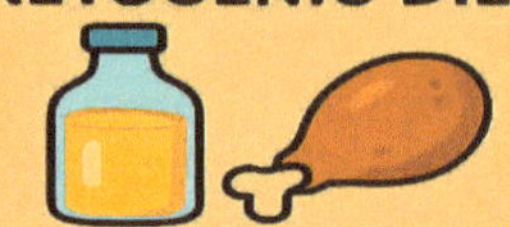

Understanding Ketogenic Ratios: What is 1:1 to 4:1?

The ketogenic diet is calculated in ratios of fat to combined protein and carbohydrate. These are expressed in ratios like 1:1, 2:1, 3:1, or 4:1.

- **1:1** = For every 1 gram of protein + carbohydrate, there is 1 gram of fat

- **2:1** = For every 1 gram of protein + carbohydrate, there are 2 grams of fat

- **3:1** = For every 1 gram of protein + carbohydrate, there are 3 grams of fat

- **4:1** = For every 1 gram of protein + carbohydrate, there are 4 grams of fat

Higher ratios like 4:1 mean more fat and stricter control on carbs and proteins. Lower ratios like 2:1 is more liberal. Most children start with a 2:1 ratio and may shift to 3:1 or 4:1 based on seizure control and tolerance.

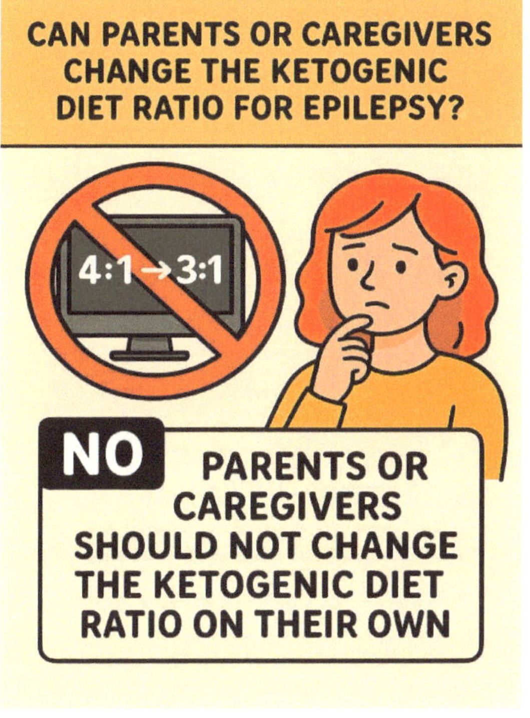

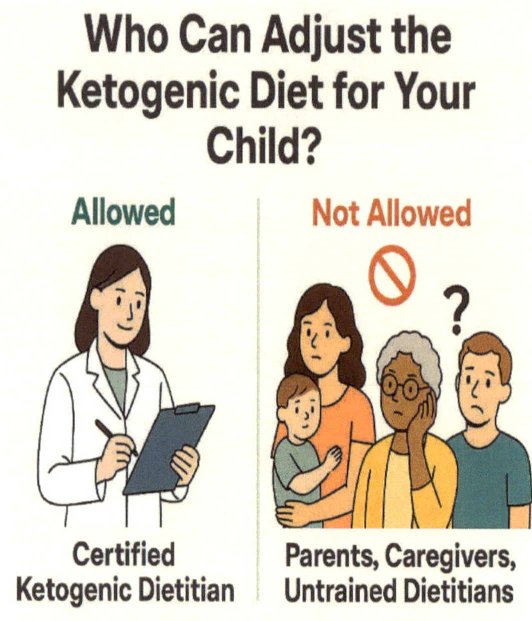

Parents or caregivers **should not change the ketogenic diet ratio** on their own when it's being used for epilepsy treatment. The **ketogenic diet for epilepsy** is a **prescribed medical nutrition therapy**, not just a low-carb lifestyle.

It's tailored to the child's age, weight, seizure type, medical history, lab values. Changing the ratio (e.g., from 4:1 to 3:1) can throw off the carefully balanced **fat-to-carb/protein** proportions needed to maintain **ketosis** which is the therapeutic state that helps control seizures.

Adjustments *can* be made, but only by a **treating team**, usually consisting of a pediatric epileptologist or a certified ketogenic dietitian.

When and Why Do Ratios Change?

Your treating team may increase or decrease the ratio depending on:

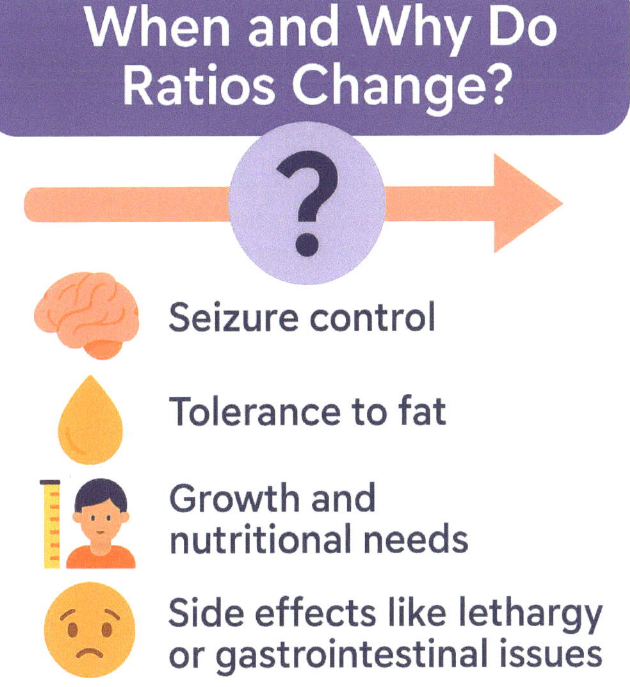

Clinical Parameters to consider Before starting Ketogenic Diet

- EEG, ECG (in some cases)
- Biochemical Parameters: liver, kidney, lipid profile, carnitine, selenium, electrolytes
- Urine Analysis: Urine test
- Anthropometry: Height, Weight, BMI

Items You Need Before Starting the Diet

- Digital food scale (0.1g accuracy)
- Measuring tools
- Ketone strips or blood monitor
- Food diary
- Blender, molds, etc.
- Supplements (multivitamin, calcium, etc.)
- Glucose gel/tablets

Four Phases of the Ketogenic Diet

Phase	Duration	Key Features
1. Carbohydrate (CHO) Washout	2–3 days	• Gradual reduction of carbohydrates • Prepares the body for ketosis
2. Initiation Phase	1-2 weeks	• Start with 2:1 fat to carb + protein ratio • Monitor ketones and side effects
3. Fine-Tuning Phase	Ongoing	• Adjust ratio (up to 4:1) • Monitor seizure control and lab values • Adapt meals/calories
4. Tapering (Weaning) Phase	After 2–3 years if effective	• Gradual reduction of fat ratio • Slow reintroduction of carbs • Requires close monitoring

Indian Food List for Different Ketogenic Diets

Food Group	Classical KD	MAD	MCT KD	LGIT
Cereals & Grains	🚫 Avoid all: rice, wheat, jowar, bajra, ragi	🚫 Avoid all: rice, roti, maida	🚫 Avoid all: grains, suji	🚫 Avoid white rice, maida, bread ✔ Allow limited whole wheat, quinoa (low GI)
Pulses & Legumes	🚫 Avoid: all dals (chana dal, masoor dal, rajma)	🚫 Avoid: heavy dals ✔ Tiny peanuts, almond flour	🚫 Avoid: lentils ✔ Limited peanut flour	✔ Allow: green moong dal, masoor dal (small quantity) 🚫 Avoid rajma, chole

(Contd.)

Food Group	Classical KD	MAD	MCT KD	LGIT
Vegetables	✔ Include: spinach, methi, lauki, tinda, broccoli, zucchini 🚫 Avoid: potato, sweet potato, yam	✔ Include: bhindi, lauki, palak 🚫 Avoid: corn, potatoes	✔ Same as Classical KD + cooked with MCT oil	✔ Include: bhindi, lauki, carrots (small amount) 🚫 Avoid: potato, sweet corn
Fruits	🚫 Avoid almost all ✔ Only small avocado portion	✔ Include small berries 🚫 Avoid banana, mango, chikoo	✔ Same berries ✔ Small fruits with MCT boost	✔ Allow: berries, apple (small), guava 🚫 Avoid: jackfruit, banana, watermelon
Milk & Dairy Products	✔ Include: paneer (full-fat), cream, ghee, cheese 🚫 Avoid skimmed milk	✔ Paneer, butter, cheese 🚫 Milk sweets	✔ Paneer, curd, fresh cream with MCT oil	✔ Homemade curd, paneer, unsweetened yogurt 🚫 Sweets made from milk

Food Group	Classical KD	MAD	MCT KD	LGIT
Meat, Fish, Eggs	✔ Include: fatty mutton, chicken (with skin), eggs, fish ⃠ Avoid breaded meats	✔ Chicken tikka, egg bhurji (dry) ⃠ Fried meats with coatings	✔ Same as Classical KD + MCT oil cooking	✔ Grilled chicken, fish, eggs ⃠ Battered or deep-fried meats
Fats & Oils	✔ Ghee, coconut oil, butter, olive oil	✔ Ghee, coconut oil, mustard oil	✔ MCT oil, coconut oil, butter	✔ Mustard oil, coconut oil, olive oil

The information provided in this table is for general guidance only and should not be considered as personalized medical or dietary advice. For a customized ketogenic diet plan tailored to your child's specific health needs, lifestyle, and goals, it is essential to consult a certified ketogenic dietitian and pediatric epileptologist. Always seek professional advice before making significant dietary changes.

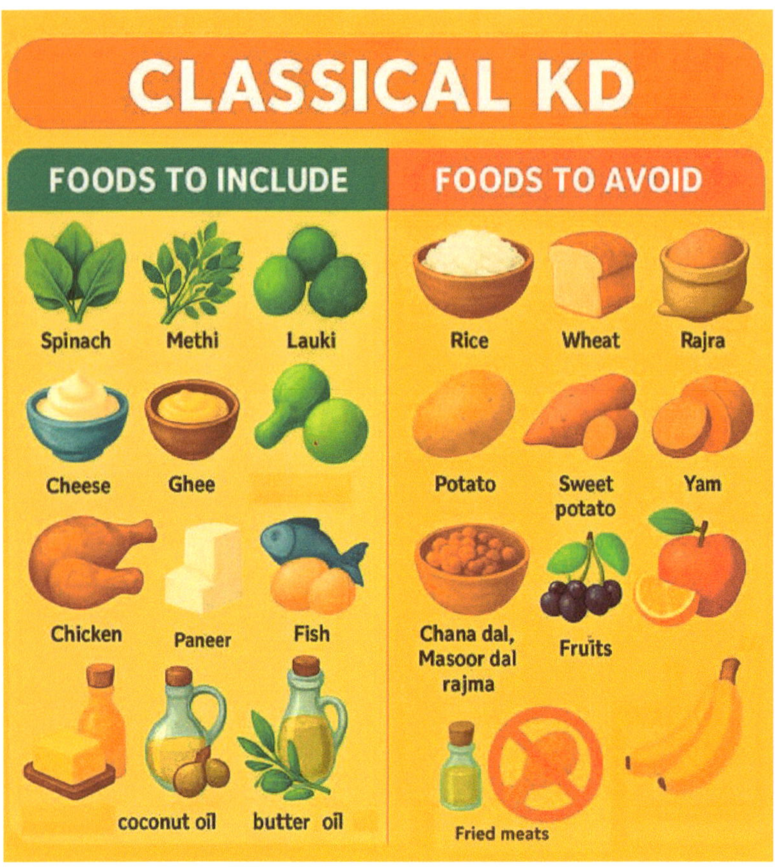
CLASSICAL KD
FOODS TO INCLUDE
FOODS TO AVOID
Spinach
Methi
Lauki
Cheese
Ghee
Chicken
Paneer
Fish
coconut oil
butter oil
Rice
Wheat
Rajra
Potato
Sweet potato
Yam
Chana dal, Masoor dal rajma
Fruits
Fried meats

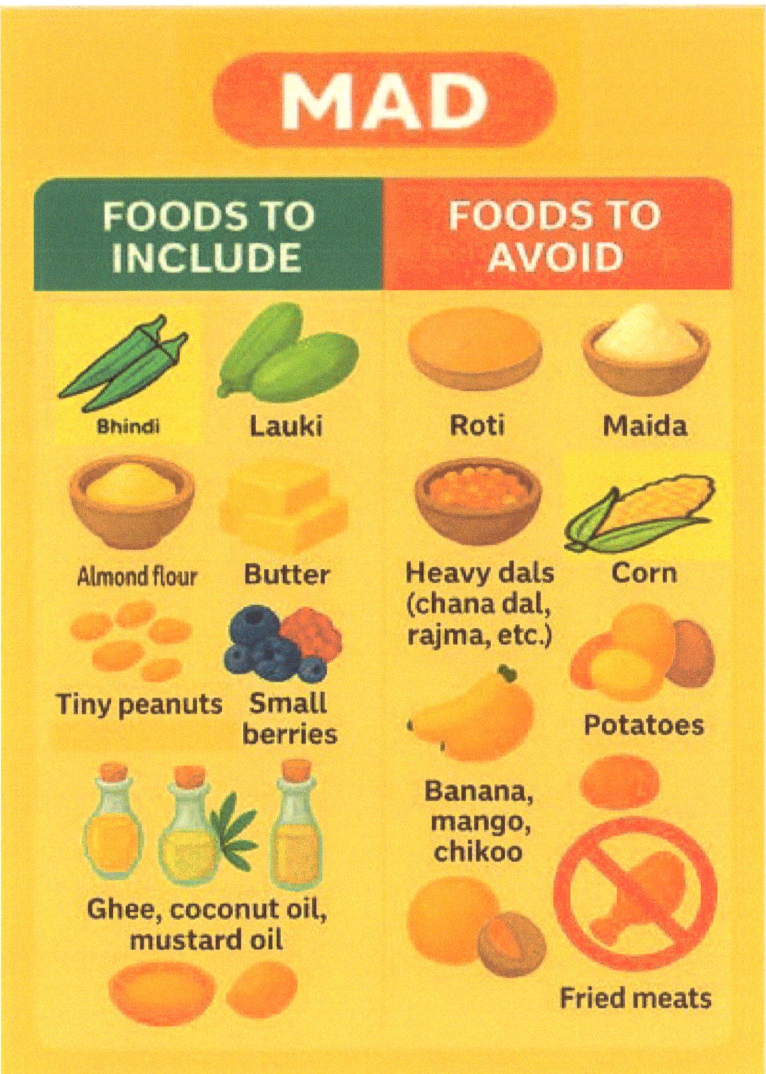
MAD
FOODS TO INCLUDE
FOODS TO AVOID
Bhindi
Lauki
Roti
Maida
Almond flour
Butter
Heavy dals (chana dal, rajma, etc.)
Corn
Tiny peanuts
Small berries
Potatoes
Ghee, coconut oil, mustard oil
Banana, mango, chikoo
Fried meats

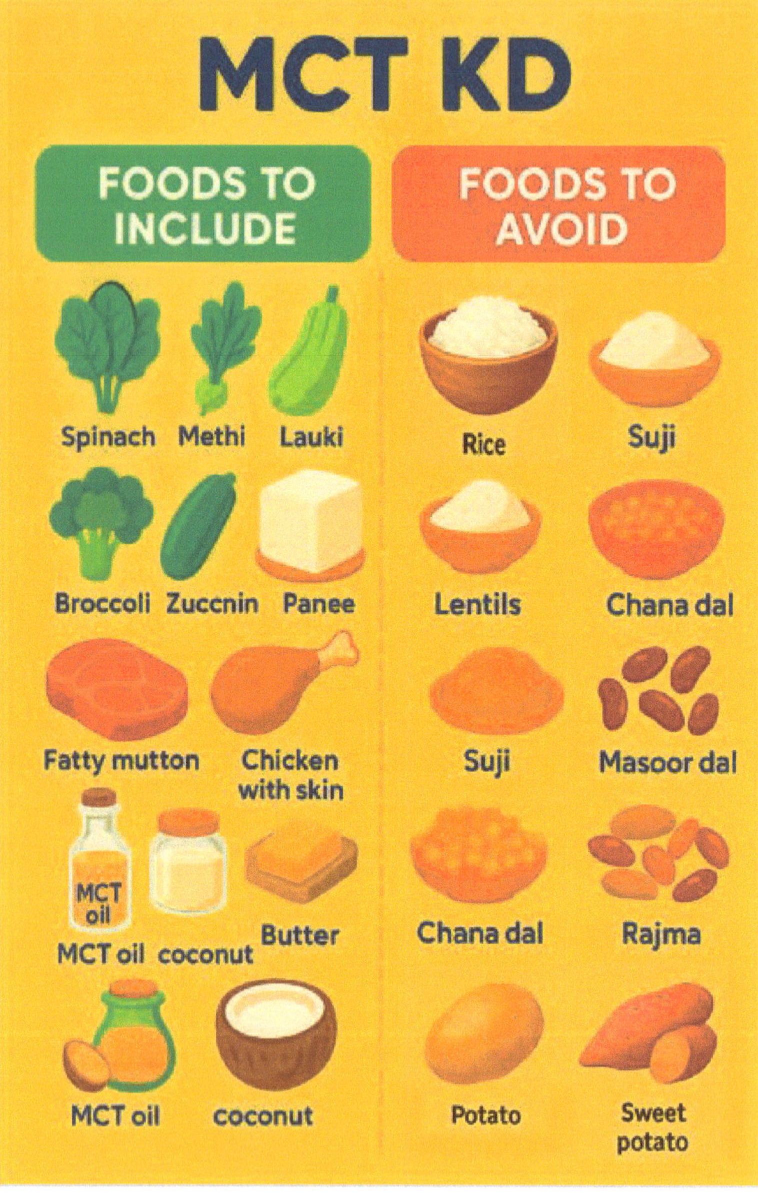
MCT KD
FOODS TO INCLUDE
FOODS TO AVOID
Spinach
Methi
Lauki
Broccoli
Zuccnin
Panee
Fatty mutton
Chicken with skin
MCT oil
MCT oil
coconut
Butter
MCT oil
coconut
Rice
Suji
Lentils
Chana dal
Suji
Masoor dal
Chana dal
Rajma
Potato
Sweet potato

LGIT

FOODS TO INCLUDE	FOODS TO AVOID

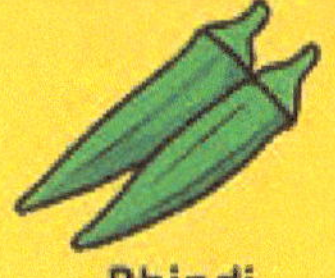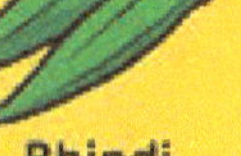 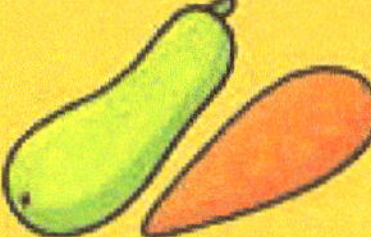 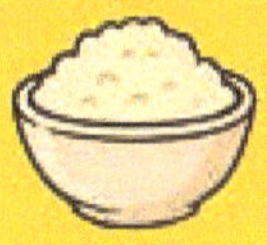 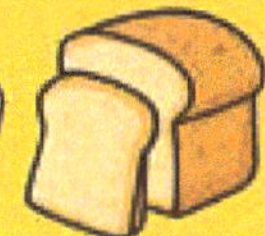

Bhindi   Carrots   White rice   Bread

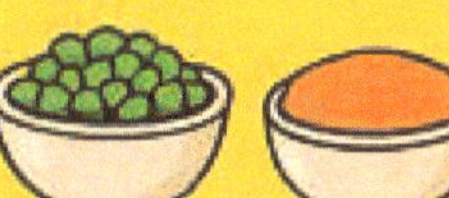 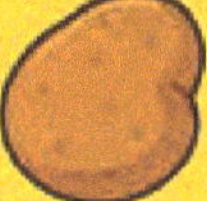 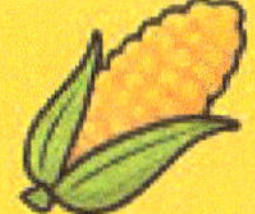

Green moong dal   Masoor dal   Apple   Potato   Sweet corn

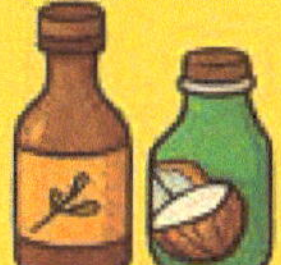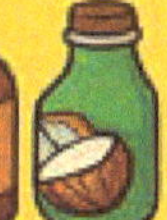 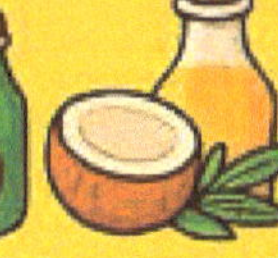 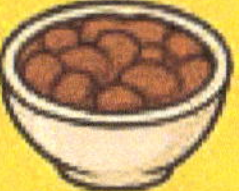 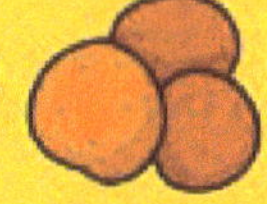

Berries   Apple   Paneer   Rajma   Chole

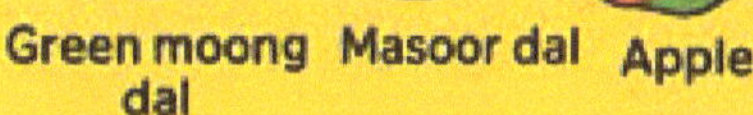 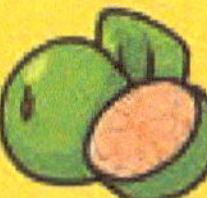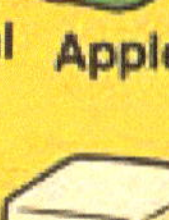 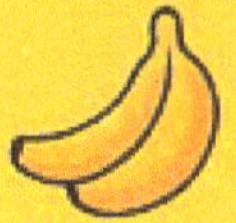 

Mustard oil   Coconut oil   Olive oil   Banana   Watermelon

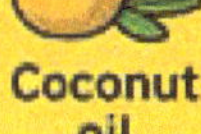 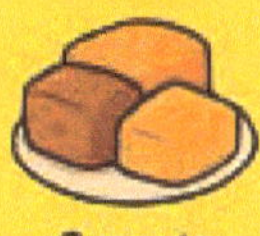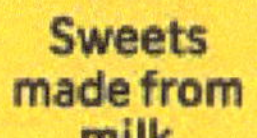 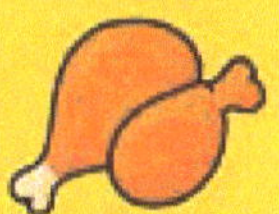

Mustard oil   Coconut oil   Olive oil   Sweets made from milk   Battered or deep-fried meats

Building a Foundation for Success

While it takes dedication, the support from pediatric epileptologist and certified keto dietician the power of preparation makes a huge difference. With every step you take—from pre-counseling to fine-tuning—you're giving your child a powerful chance at better health and seizure control.

Chapter 4

MONITORING AND MAINTAINING
THE KETOGENIC DIET

Routine Monitoring

Once your child is on the ketogenic diet, regular monitoring is essential to ensure safety, effectiveness, and proper growth. Monitoring typically includes:

- Ketone levels (via urine or blood)
- Blood glucose levels
- Weight and growth tracking
- Blood tests: lipid profile, liver/kidney function, electrolytes, carnitine, selenium
- Seizure diary to assess frequency, severity, and triggers

Clinic Visits

Children on the ketogenic diet should visit the dietitian and pediatric neurologist every 1–3 months initially. During these visits:

- Growth is monitored
- Diet adjustments are made

- Lab results are reviewed
- Parents can ask questions and review progress

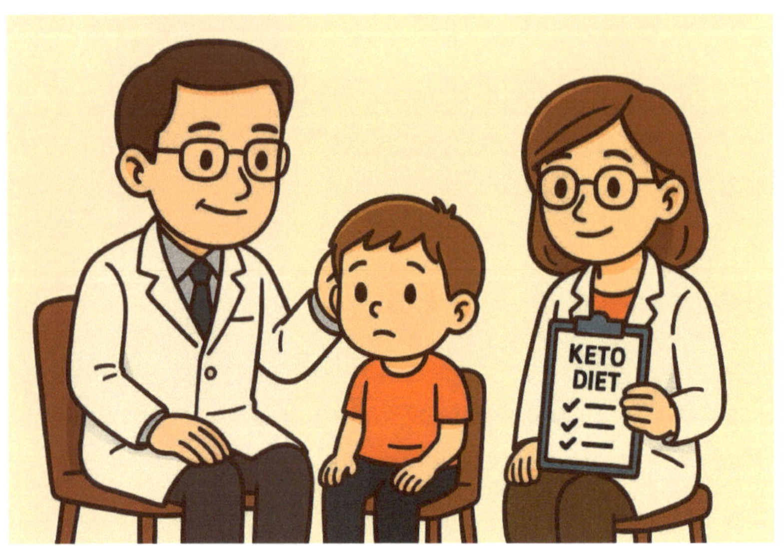

Managing Illness and Emergencies

During illness (fever, diarrhea, vomiting), maintaining ketosis can be challenging. You may need to:

- Switch to simple, high-fat tolerated meals
- Monitor hydration and ketone levels more frequently
- Use glucose gel for suspected hypoglycemia
- Contact your care team for guidance

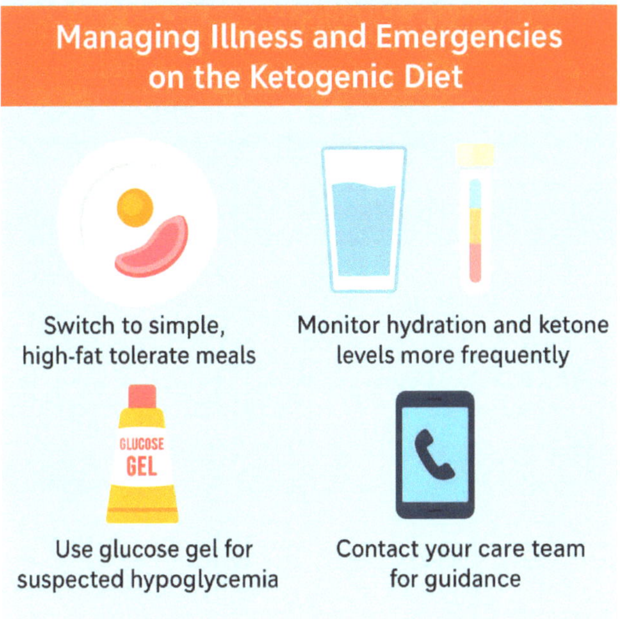

Challenges During Ketogenic Diet Initiation – For Caregivers

Problem	Why It Happens	What You Can Do
Low Blood Sugar (Hypoglycemia)	Sudden drop in carbs before full fat-adaptation	• Monitor blood sugar • Start diet gradually • Use glucose tablets if advised
Dehydration & Electrolyte Imbalance	Ketosis causes water and salt loss	• Give plenty of fluids • Use electrolyte-rich broths or supplements if needed

(Contd.)

Problem	Why It Happens	What You Can Do
Constipation	Low fiber & fluids	• Include keto-safe fiber foods (flax, zucchini) • Increase fluids • Use laxatives if prescribed
Loss of Appetite / Nausea	Fat-heavy meals can feel too rich	• Serve smaller, frequent meals • Offer variety • Be patient — it usually passes
Fatigue / Irritability ('Keto Flu')	Body adjusting to fat metabolism	• Let child rest • Stay hydrated • Reassure: symptoms are temporary
Seizures Worsen Initially	Not all respond quickly or diet needs adjustment	• Keep logs • Notify keto team immediately • Possible ratio tweak or other changes

Adjusting the Diet Over Time

As your child grows, the diet will evolve:

- Calories and protein requirements change

- Food preferences may shift

- Side effects may appear and need management

- Seizure frequency may guide ratio adjustments

How to Check Urine Ketones at Home

For Children on the Ketogenic Diet for Epilepsy and Seizure Control

✓ What You Need

- Urine ketone test strips (available at pharmacies)

- A clean container (optional)

- Access to the color chart (on the strip bottle)

- Timer (or a phone)

📝 Step-by-Step Guide

1. Wash hands – Hygiene is important before testing.

2. Collect urine sample:

   - Option A: Let the child urinate directly onto the strip.

   - Option B: Collect urine in a clean cup and dip the strip.

3. Dip the strip into the urine for about 1–2 seconds.

4. Hold the strip flat and wait for 15–60 seconds (follow the strip brand's instructions).

5. Compare the color on the strip with the chart on the test strip bottle.

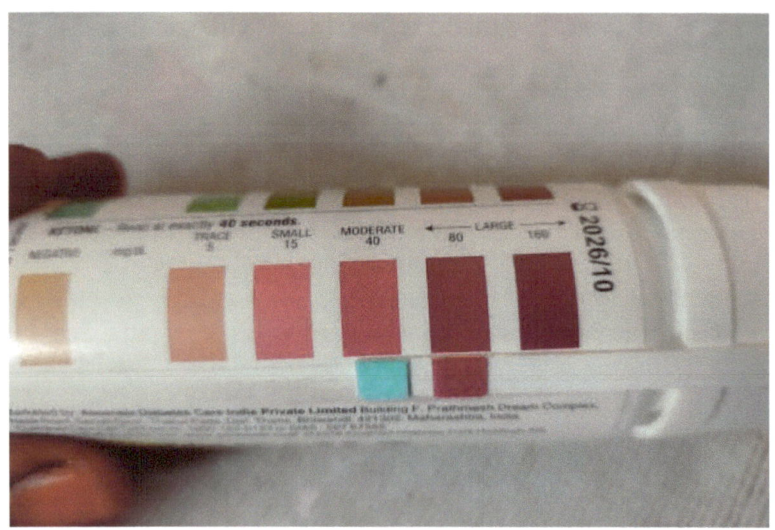

Urine Ketone Test Strip

🎯 What Are You Looking For?

Color on Strip	Ketone Level	What It Means
No change	Negative	No ketones detected
Light pink	Trace	Early-stage ketosis — acceptable during diet initiation
Medium pink	Small to Moderate	Ideal ketosis for seizure control
Dark purple	Large	Deep ketosis — monitor hydration and symptoms

⚠️ Watch for These Signs

- Vomiting
- Drowsiness

- Confusion
- Breathing changes
- Irritability or fatigue

☐→ If these symptoms appear along with high ketones (4++ or 160 mg/dL), inform your pediatric neurologist or dietitian right away.

💡 Tips for Parents

- Test thrice at the same time daily (usually morning, afternoon and night).
- Keep a log of ketone levels for your dietitian or pediatric neurologist.
- Make sure your child stays well-hydrated.

How long will it take for Ketogenic Diet to show its effect in reducing seizures?

The **ketogenic diet can begin to show its effects on epilepsy in children within days to weeks**, but the **full benefits may take a few months** to become clear.

Here's a general timeline:

⏱ 1–2 Weeks: Early Effects

- Some children experience a **reduction in seizure frequency within the first few days to two weeks.**
- This is more common in children who are very responsive to the diet.

- **Ketosis usually begins within 3–10 days** if the diet is followed strictly.

📅 1–3 Months: Monitoring Phase

- Most medical teams do a **trial period of 2–3 months** to evaluate effectiveness.

- If significant seizure reduction (often ≥50%) is seen, the diet may be continued long term.

⧗ 6 Months and Beyond

- For children who respond well, seizure control can **continue to improve over time**.

- Some may become seizure-free or reduce their medication load gradually under supervision.

🔄 Key Things to Remember

- **Not every child responds** to the diet, but about **30–60%** see meaningful seizure reduction.

- Regular follow-up with the **keto team** (pediatric neurologist + certified keto dietitian) is essential to adjust the plan and check for side effects.

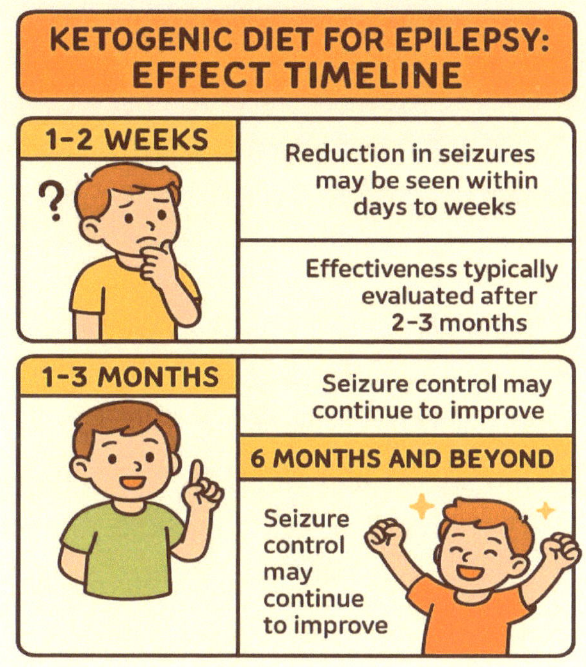

What is Honeymoon effect of Ketogenic Diet?

The **"honeymoon effect"** of the ketogenic diet in epilepsy refers to an initial period of significant improvement in seizure control soon after starting the diet, followed by a **partial or complete return of seizures** over time.

What Happens During the Honeymoon Effect?

- **Initial Response (First few weeks to months):** Many children experience a **dramatic reduction or complete cessation of seizures** shortly after starting the ketogenic diet. This is often seen as a "honeymoon phase" where the diet seems highly effective.

- **Later Phase (Several months in):** For some, the effectiveness diminishes, and seizures may begin to return or increase in frequency/intensity. This doesn't mean the diet has failed but indicates a **plateau or need for adjustments** (e.g., ratio changes, food compliance, or adjunct therapies).

🔍 Possible Reasons for the Honeymoon Effect

- **Initial metabolic shift** leads to higher ketone levels, rapidly altering brain chemistry and reducing excitability.

- **Adaptation over time**: The brain may become less responsive to ketones, or dietary adherence may wane.

- **Disease progression**: Some underlying epilepsies are progressive and may naturally worsen over time.

📖 Clinical Insight

A study by Kang HC et al. (2005) noted that **seizure control is most significant in the first 3 months** of initiating the ketogenic diet, after which the effect may decline in some children. Continuous monitoring and dietary adjustments are crucial to maintain benefits.

Peer Influence and How to Overcome It

Managing a strict ketogenic diet for a child with drug-resistant epilepsy (DRE) can feel isolating at times. One of the biggest challenges parents face isn't just the diet itself — it's **peer influence**. Well-meaning friends, family, teachers, and even other parents may unintentionally pressure you to loosen restrictions, offer alternative treatments, or question the diet's necessity.

Understanding **how peer influence works** — and developing strategies to **overcome it** — is essential for staying consistent and confident in your child's care plan.

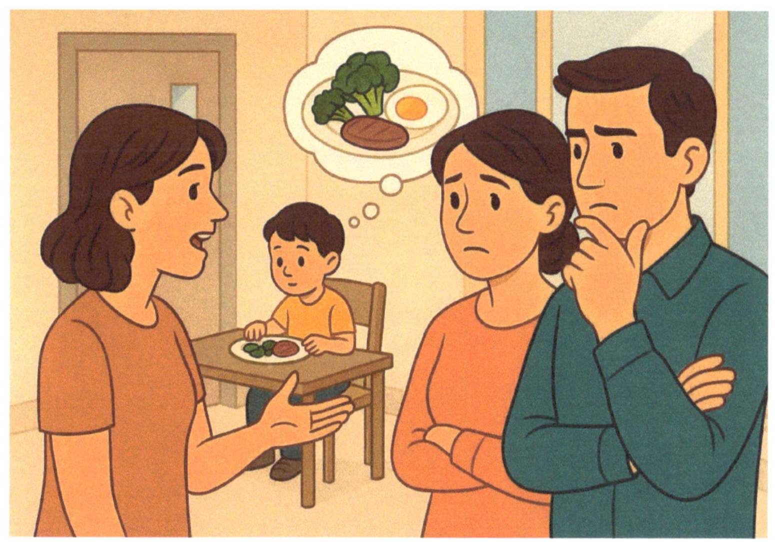

How Peer Influence Shows Up

- **Family Gatherings**: Relatives may encourage "just one treat" or say "one time won't hurt."

- **Social Events**: Other parents may offer non-keto snacks without understanding the medical importance.

- **School Environment**: Teachers or staff might not realize the seriousness of dietary compliance.

- **Online Communities**: Other parents in epilepsy groups might push alternative therapies that conflict with keto.

- **Healthcare Settings**: Occasionally, even non-specialist doctors or dietitians may question the strictness of a therapeutic ketogenic diet.

Why Peer Influence Can Be So Powerful

- Desire to **fit in** or not seem "difficult."
- Fear of being labeled as "overprotective" or "extreme."
- Emotional fatigue — wanting your child to feel "normal" during social events.
- Doubt creeping in when trusted people question your choices.

Strategies for Overcoming Peer Influence

1. Know Your 'Why' Clearly

Have a crystal-clear understanding of why your child is on the ketogenic diet. This is not a fad — it is a **medically prescribed therapy** to manage a serious condition. Keep a mental list (or a note on your phone) of the improvements you've seen.

"We're not just doing keto for lifestyle reasons. This is medical nutrition therapy, as vital as any medication."

2. Educate Your Circle

Provide short, easy-to-understand explanations when necessary. You don't need to get into deep science unless you want to, but a simple statement like:

"His brain needs a special kind of fuel to prevent seizures. Breaking the diet could cause a medical emergency."

3. Set Clear Boundaries (Politely)

Practice responses you can use when someone challenges you:

- *"Thanks for offering, but we'll bring his own food."*
- *"I appreciate your concern, but we're following his neurologist's plan very carefully."*
- *"It's not about preference; it's about his health and safety."*

4. Build a Support Network

Find other parents who are also managing keto for epilepsy. Having even one or two people who truly get it can make all the difference. Online forums, local epilepsy foundations, and hospital programs often have parent support groups.

5. Plan Ahead

For events or trips:

- Bring keto-friendly versions of common treats.
- Talk to hosts, teachers, or organizers ahead of time.
- Have a prepared statement ready for those curious about your child's food.

6. Trust Yourself

Remember: *You are your child's best advocate.*

No one else will understand your child's needs as you do. Trust in the medical team, your experience, and your intuition.

7. Focus on the Bigger Picture

Every time you resist social pressure, you're investing in your child's long-term health, cognitive development, and seizure control. It's worth the occasional awkward moment or hard conversation.

Peer influence is real, but it doesn't have to derail your child's therapy. With preparation, confidence, and support, you can stay true to the ketogenic plan — and protect your child's health above all else.

You're not being difficult. You're being **brave** and **wise**. And you're not alone.

Support Systems and Communication

Educating family members, school staff, and caregivers is essential. Provide:

- Written meal plans
- Emergency instructions (e.g., what to do for hypoglycemia)
- Explanation of the diet's importance
- Inclusion in daily routines

FREQUENTLY ASKED QUESTIONS (FAQS) BY PARENTS AND CAREGIVERS ON KETOGENIC DIET AT OUR CLINIC

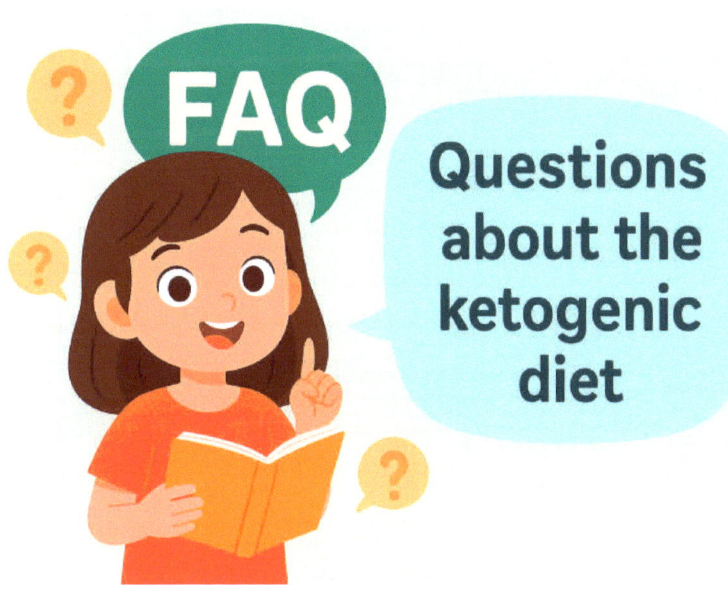

Question	Answer
1. What is the ketogenic diet?	It is a high-fat, low-carbohydrate, adequate-protein diet used as a medical nutrition therapy for epilepsy.
2. How does it help in epilepsy?	It produces ketones that alter brain metabolism and reduce seizure activity.
3. Can the diet cure epilepsy?	It may significantly reduce or eliminate seizures, but it is not a guaranteed cure.
4. Is it safe for all children?	Yes, it is safe for children but should be monitored closely under supervision of certified keto dietician and pediatric epileptologist.
5. Do we need hospital admission to start?	Not always. Home initiation is common unless your pediatric epileptologist recommends otherwise.
6. How long should the diet be followed?	Usually 2–3 years, but it's individualized and depends on child's seizure control and needs. Conditions like GLUT 1 Deficiency Syndrome and in PDH Deficiency Disorder Ketogenic Diet should be continued lifelong.

Question	Answer
7. Can Indian vegetarian meals be adapted?	Yes, with proper planning to maintain the ratio under supervision of certified keto dietician.
8. Can we include ghee and butter?	Yes, they are excellent fat sources in ketogenic meals.
9. What are good Indian keto ingredients?	Coconut, paneer, cream, almond flour, cauliflower, and nuts.
10. How is a keto meal planned?	By calculating fat, protein, and carbs precisely for each meal by certified keto dietician.
11. What's the most common starting ratio?	2:1 ratio is commonly started in children.
12. Can we give fruits?	Only a few like avocado or berries in small amounts, depending on carb limits. Other fruits in form of milkshakes using high fat milk carefully planned by certified keto dietician.
13. Is milk allowed?	Regular milk is limited; cream or diluted coconut milk, soya milk or almond milk is preferred.

(Contd.)

Question	Answer
14. How is ketosis monitored?	Through urine ketone strips or blood ketone meters.
15. What do high ketone levels mean?	It usually indicates effective ketosis but should be monitored for side effects.
16. What are signs of low blood sugar?	Fatigue, shakiness, confusion, irritability.
17. How to treat low sugar?	Give glucose gel or small amount of fast-acting carbohydrate under supervision.
18. Can we send keto meals to school?	Yes, with careful prep and communication with school staff.
19. Can grandparents follow the diet too?	It's for epilepsy treatment only. Seniors must consult a doctor separately.
20. Can it affect growth?	Sometimes. That's why growth is closely monitored.
21. What if my child gets bored of the meals?	Work with your dietitian to diversify recipes and textures.
22. Can it cause constipation?	Yes, but it can be managed with fiber, fluids, and mild laxatives.
23. Can we use sugar-free products?	No, some sweeteners affect ketosis, consult your clinical dietician for the alternatives.

Question	Answer
24. Can it be done during festivals?	Yes, but needs careful planning and substitute meals under supervision of trained keto dietician.
25. Is there any religious concern?	Most foods can be adjusted for cultural and religious needs.
26. Are supplements necessary?	Yes, multivitamins, calcium, and selenium are usually prescribed.
27. What is the cost of the diet?	It varies but may increase grocery bills due to specialty foods.
28. Can it be done with other therapies?	Yes. It is often combined with medications and therapies.
29. Can a picky eater follow the diet?	Yes, with creativity and slow transitions.
30. Is it covered by insurance?	In India, most insurance doesn't cover dietary therapy yet.
31. Can I find keto foods in Indian stores?	Yes, many items like paneer, cream, ghee, coconut are easily available.
32. What is keto flu?	A temporary state of fatigue, irritability, or headache as the body adjusts.
33. Can I prepare meals in advance?	Yes, meal prepping helps a lot in managing time.
34. Are restaurant foods allowed?	Usually not. It's hard to calculate macros accurately.

(Contd.)

Question	Answer
35. What oil is best?	Coconut oil, olive oil, ghee are excellent sources of fat.
36. Can I stop the diet suddenly?	No. It must be tapered off under medical supervision.
37. Is Modified Atkins different?	Yes. It's less strict and sometimes used after keto.
38. What if seizures increase on keto?	Inform your pediatric neurologist and dietician. Adjustments may be needed.
39. Can my child play sports?	Yes. Energy may improve after initial adjustment.
40. What if my child vomits a meal?	Contact the treating team. Maintain hydration and ketone tracking.
41. Can this be done in rural areas?	Yes, consult your clinical dietician who will help you out in planning meal based on local food availability.
42. How often are labs done?	Every 3–6 months or as per the pediatric neurologist and dietician's advice.
43. Can I use almond or coconut flour?	Yes, they are commonly used low-carb flours.

Question	Answer
44. Are there support groups in India?	Yes, online and hospital-based support is growing.
45. How do I explain the diet to relatives?	Use written resources or invite them to a dietitian session.
46. Can epilepsy come back after stopping keto?	Possibly. That's why tapering is slow and supervised.
47. Can my child fast for religious reasons?	Discuss with your pediatric neurologist; fasting may not be safe.
48. Can I use Ayurveda with keto?	Only under medical supervision, to avoid interaction.
49. What if we make a mistake in meals?	Mistakes happen. Correct and continue with guidance.
50. Can the child travel while on keto?	Yes. Pack meals, monitor ketones, and maintain routine.

REFERENCES

1. International League Against Epilepsy. Available from: https://www.ilae.org/

2. Kossoff EH, Zupec-Kania BA, Amark PE, Ballaban-Gil KR, Bergqvist AGC, Blackford R, et al. Optimal clinical management of children receiving the ketogenic diet: Recommendations of the International Ketogenic Diet Study Group. *Epilepsia*. 2009 Feb;50(2):304–17.

3. Neal EG, Chaffe H, Schwartz RH, Lawson MS, Edwards N, Fitzsimmons G, et al. The ketogenic diet for the treatment of childhood epilepsy: a randomised controlled trial. *Lancet Neurol*. 2008 Jun;7(6):500–6.

4. Kang HC, Chung DE, Kim DW, Kim HD. Early- and late-onset complications of the ketogenic diet for intractable epilepsy. Epilepsia. 2004 Sep;45(9):1116–23.